I0758194

WEIGHT

IN

GOLD

Heidi Kaplan

First published 2020
ISBN: 9798851042416

All Rights Reserved
Heidi Kaplan ©2020
Front cover photograph Heidi Kaplan ©2020
Additional illustrative work Meek ©2020

Heidi has asserted her moral right to be identified as the author of this work in accordance with the Copyright, Designs and Patents Act 1988.

An Inherit The Earth Publication © 2020
In conjunction with Amazon

Edited by Meek 2020

My stepfather Robert Stromberg, who always had a pad and black biro to jot down his writing. And always encouraged my songwriting from the very beginning. He would be very proud to see this book.

Heidi. x

Editor's Preface –

I met Heidi through our collaborative writing project For The Many Not The Few. This is Heidi's first published book. Her poems and lyrics deal with genuine issues in her life. I was greatly inspired by her words while compiling and editing her book. Heidi writes from personal experienced, from her heart and from a life worth living. She doesn't shy away from what confronts her. She bares her raw soul. She's a brave writer. Avail yourself to her narrative.

CT Meek
April 2020.

Contents

Weight in Gold.

Autumn leaves were falling

The air was fresh and cold

The moon was full and I felt too alone

So I took a drive to your house

We sat and talked til dawn

Good friend I think you're worth your weight in gold

Told you when I met you

I like the way you smile

Turn any corner and I will meet you there

Spent all these years hoping for a saint to reappear

Well good friend I think you're worth your weight in gold

So don't try to fool me with all your potent talk

About setting out to sea some day

Cos you know you'll only miss us

And start heading home again

So promise that you'll always stay

Cos good friend I think you're worth your weight in gold

And our secrets will watch all our hopes unfold.

Beneath The Surface

I've worked for people with serious money
With little else to show to you
Once you've toured the house
No humility or Grace
Charity or respect or even humour
For those who pass through their doors.

We are just replaceable bodies
Workhorse commodities
Minimum wages and be happy with that
You're lucky to be here
Please leave your shoes at the door
Oh and here is the list of your multiple chores

Why does money change you?
Or were they always so shallow and mean?
Questions that you cannot answer
Sweep it under the carpet and it all goes away
Empty values and silver decanters

Everything feels ugly with decay
It's not a home
Not as you'd describe
The chairs sit stifled
The sofas Baron
The artworks colourless hues
I'd rather have a shack made of wood
Than this mansion with its heart of stone.

Good Grief

Death changes everything
We are left with our ineptitude
And to consider one's fate
Like a store bought sweater that you soon learn to hate

Because it never stopped itching
And was always too short
Like my time with you I suppose.
When you are young the world seems so large
Your laughter permeates the air
And time moves so slow
But that's changed now
Time flies by
But the missing you feels endless
Like a sentence I'm destined to fulfil
Always alone and just waiting
To meet with you again on the other side

Death makes you tired
It's too easy to quit
All numbing and sure fire self-pity
It can feel oddly principled
Like it knows where it's going and that's
Nowhere fast
Enough already!

Eye Of A Needle.

Through the eye of a needle
I see many, many things
Darkness and light
In varying degrees
Hard men pimps with hearts of stone
Washed up beauties already too old

Tales of love and tales of truth
Tales of some cruel and reckless brute who really
Listens and who really cares
You've got money in your pocket
For a second class fare
You've got money in your pocket
For a second class fare

I hope for pastures fresh and green
And I hope you keep your garden clean
But time trips us up
And closes the door
I think we're all worth so much more
Yes I think we're all worth so much more

Through the eye of a needle
I see many, many things
Long dusty roads with no one at home
Mothers and fathers watching out for their sons
Shell shocked heroes lie in bed with their guns

Dreams of war and dreams of peace
Dreams of lust on warm satin sheets
I think we've all got something to lose
So I'll just stay home and sing the blues

I'll just stay home and sing .....
The Blues.

Stoners United.
Life without a filter can be sullenly dull
Filled with obligatory tenderness
And heavy brown curtains
Keeping out light
Dusty shelves filled with memories
A chapter from a marathon dream

That's what dope does
It colours the walls
And makes one more interested
In the mundane everyday chores
The chiming of a clock keeping rhythm
The dainty song of blackbirds keeping score

That's what I say anyway
Nothing chemical or nasty or vile
Just some herbs and a lighter
And a contented smile

Think I will construct a multi-coloured,
Multi-textured, multi-layered magnificent
Lasagne in short while!

Say Cheese.

Leave A Light On.
This is the story about a friend I used to know
He had troubled times and never let his feelings show
Then one day he gave the game away
Cleared his throat so I could hear him say

Chorus: Leave a light on in heaven for me
Cos I could be you and you could be me
Leave a light on I want you to see that I love you,
I love you, I love you
You mean the world to me

Well he started travelling and the road became his home
So we lost touch, he'd just forgotten how to phone
I knew he'd be okay
As the months turned into years
No news was good news
He's only conquering his fears

What now I hear? He's gotten married
She had his child,
Seemed so strange he was always free, my wild Fire

I felt cheated, kinda saddened and forlorn
So I wrote this song and hoped that he might sing along
Leave a light on in heaven for me
Cos I could be you and you could be me
Leave alight on
I want you to see that I love you, I love you,
Love you, you mean the world to me

Now that was years ago and I haven't heard a word
But I still dream of him
I know it sounds absurd

Time gives you distance
And lots of time for regret

Now that old first love is the one I can't forget
So leave a light on in heaven for me
Cos I could be you
And you could be me
Leave a light on I want you to see
That I love you, I love you, I love you
You mean the world to me
This is a story about a friend I used to know.

Home To Me.

Got my paper, got my pen
Searching for some motivation
Whilst thinking about my dedication
Do I really need to go through this again?
I feel no direction, or free flow
Like Blind Man's bluff
Or finding cake crumbs in the snow
Do I really need to go through this again?
I do it cos I need it
I do it cos I love it
I do it cos it takes me home to me

In the past it came so quick,
When I was younger fresh and true
I thought I wrote some graceful wit
With a definite destination
I can blame my lack of education
Do I really need to go through this again?

Just write as it comes a friend suggests
And don't overthink it too much
I'm listening in, yet tuning out,
Whilst heading straight back to my room
Do I really need to go through this again?
I do it cos I need it
I do it cos I love it
I do it cos it takes me home to me

Another day rolled out some simple lines
I'm feeling better and like I'm not a waste of time
A poignant pause was all it took
Back in the rhythm just like an old familiar book
Do I really need to go through this again?

The end is near I'm glad to say,
This pen and paper have painted many shades of grey
A new built horizon meets the shore
I'll close this now and then I'll be back to write some more
Do I really need to go through this again?
I do it cos I need it
I do it cos I love it
I do it cos it takes me home to me.

Song For Mona.

My funny older sister, an original wild child
With a natural orange streak running through her hair
Marked to be different from an early age
The friendship she gave me could never be replaced
We made up our own language to our disgrace
We jumped on the bed and laughed til we cried
We decorated our walls with pop stars of fame
Dreamt of them all through the night
And then she learnt to play the sweetest guitar
And I'd sing with her, my biggest delight
She played it at school, and she sang like a bird
Fourteen and up on the stage alone
The audience was silent as they observed
I was so proud, she had made me cry
These memories can never die
We sang and played songs till our throats felt dry
We sounded so happy and free
Our little escape from the world outside
This was our world in harmony
Then tragedy hit,
Her mind disturbed by thoughts so absurd and cruel
She didn't talk for several months
And drugs became her sharpest tool
Her body was frozen in time
The doctors helped as much as they could
While I just died inside
She's never got better, my sadness remained
Her passion and abilities for music had become a shadow
From the past
Then I started to write just on my own
She knew that and thought that I was good
My vocals sounded fine
But my biggest regret was that my finger picking sister was gone

I loved her so much
We were so very alike
Fire signs right from the start
I dedicate this song to you
Throw your arrows straight to my heart.

Free To Fly.
I heard a sweet bird singing high up on your fence today,
I recognised her melody, and she
Don't care much today,
I want to be just like her soaring
Free against your skies,
I want to be just like her, free to
Roam and free to fly.

I heard that sweet bird flew today
To a green and distant land,
No suitcase did she carry,
For she knew I'd understand
I want to be just like her soaring
Free against your skies,
I want to be just like her, free to
Roam and free to fly.

She gave me inspiration to find another road,
Except my resignation, my heart's already flown,
I send you this invitation, just follow in her mode
I sense there is no reason for this song or for this rhyme
It's just this restless feeling that we all get time to time
I want to be just like her soaring
Free against your skies
I want to be just like her free to
Roam and free to fly.

American Folk Song.
What did I teach you when you
Were so young to make you so bitter as to carry a gun?
And what can I teach you now that you're so old?
No Star Spangled Banner and your children so bold
I don't hear your preacher man
I'm gonna learn as much as I can

There's no hesitation, I hope you can hear
I don't want my children to be poisoned with fear
We're all on one world, moving incredibly slow
So wake up or shape up we reap what we sow
I don't want to hear your preacher man
I want to learn just as much as I can

Well here come the Twenties, I know we can cope
With wages and changes yet still have some hope
For magical things to have meaning at last
Machines are damn quick but they don't have a past
Look what they did to your preacher man
I'm gonna learn as I much as I can

What did I teach you when you were so young
To make you so bitter as to carry a gun?
And what can I teach you now that you are so old
No Star Spangled Banner and your children so bold.

The Waiting Room.
Sitting here waiting
I'm always waiting
Waiting for the show to begin
Where are the players
They haven't turned up
Looks like the poets have all gone home too
Their scrambled words fall silent
Recited to themselves instead

I'll seek solace in Nature
She won't let me down
I'll wait for spring instead
The blossoms will show me their colours
As "Magnolia you sweet thing," plays on in my head

Lying here witting
Over thinking the facts
Waiting for dreams to come true
Happiness waits on the other side
Strength and virtue stand by her too
I'll open this door to let them in
Then with gratitude I can finally rest

I've always been waiting
Waiting for fire, excitement or love
Making my own entertainment
Like & witches brew
Waiting for &answers
Waiting for truth
Waiting for you

Untitled.

The Queen of cold indifference
(Is not a woman you'd warm to)
Has washed her hands of you
You shall not be needed after all
Your skills are required elsewhere
Go shine your light and gather friends
You'll need all you can get in this fight

Do you seek justice or vengeance my friend?
I think not, not in this lifetime
Anyhow, the weary have arrived a little bruised and torn
We will find our escape, that one true song
That we will sing til our hearts have healed
And your Queen of cold indifference is buried
Deep within her hooded shroud
Her anguish and hostility revealed

So burn your love light brightly
Dont sit around and linger
Make a difference and shout it loud
No jealous muses needed
Believe in magic and all within will turn towards your light
And your Queen of cold indifference will vanish with the night.

Invisible In Beige.
I've applied to Tesco for a chance
To sit upon a till and chart
The many wholesome faces
Of my local rendezvous

I need a job that's easy
Not too hard upon the back
Where I can fantasise that I'm someone else
Where they will definitely cut me some slack

I will scribble my poems when I want to
When something shiny catches my eye
Or I see a handsome loved-up couple
Making out in aisle five

Now I just hope that they will want me
And that I can manage their damned machine
No more complications
Pulling at the heart strings

I want to work at Tesco
Invisible in beige
My glory days are over
Insurance for my pre-paid grave.

Love Stuff.
Misinformed and outta touch
Too hot to handle
When you love too much
Silly and foolish with longing and wile
Imagine the taste of his beautiful smile

Take it slow don't over obsess
He'll call you back when he's ready
Clean your room or wash the car
Don't wait around and mope as
This desire infiltrates everything

Now I choose to wear much
Brighter clothes see me, see me, see me!
No more drab and black or grey
Fitted right to show some hip
He'll pull me tight and we'll fuck all night
All this lust must find its outlet

But does he feel the same as me?
Does he watch the clock and cancel his friends
In the hope that you are free?
I watch his every twitch
His eyebrows
And his heart
Hoping that I might read him
So that I'm alw1ys prepared
And ready to pounce
This Lioness is restless.

Coming In Blue.
My time is coming
I've had enough of this shit
I will be free and single
Not attached like a stone

I will sing triumphantly
I've served my sentence now
I choose life as the t-shirt
And not hard labour

I've weathered a storm
Where nobody else got wet
They won't go when I go
Mr Stevie Wonder poetically said

I have only two purposes
To Laugh and to Love
And to be loved in return
I feel worn out
Unreciprocated
I'll sit here and rest
And write away the coming in blue.

Wishing Well.

Sometimes I wish I'd been somebody else
Someone less painful, prettier and free
From all of these thoughts and contemplative dreams
Someone more glamorous with the right amount of edge
Sometimes these thoughts whirl around in my head

Sometimes I wish that I'd travelled more
Sought adventure and climbed higher
That everything down here looked tiny and bright
A perfect picture framed by a brilliant blue sky

Sometimes I realise that I've always been true
I cannot pretend or declare that I'm fickle and awkward
Bound to believe that the best thing
About me is bound to be you

Sometimes I wish that I just didn't care about family fortune
And fates
That I did not think so profoundly, just lighten up
And let it be
To step away from the danger; to be floating away to be free.

Depression: A Mood Disorder.
So whaddaya y'all do?
Ignore it on a half decent day
Roll it away in a handful of joints
Swallow it down with some heavy gulps
Or take notice and divert all known traffic?
I told you, walk around the hole in the ground
Don't fall into the well like a jerk
Reason with your mate and pull yourself together
Great lyrics like "Behind A Painted Smile"
And "Mona Lisa"
Had the highway blues you can tell by the way she smiles
Say it all
Be kind
Be patient
Be reasonable
All the well-meaning quotations
Magnify the weight of the issue
Distraction is the vital key here
Writing helps me to escape
And not to dwell too long
To forget and recharge
So thankful for these small pleasures.

Momma's Cookin'.
One day when I went walking
I saw this baby boy
Well I knew that boy would make me
One mean baby toy
Well one night he came calling
Knockin on my back door
I knew he'd break his Momma's heart
Cos he don't come home no more
See he was good at foolin'
And I was torn apart
I waited there every single day
But he kept me in the dark oh Lord,
Oh, Lord

Well I believed in patience
And he believed in sin
He puffed away every single day
But I guessed where he'd been
He's gone for Momma's Cookin'
And he's gone for Momma's wine
I knew I'd been the foolish one
To think that he'd be all mine,
All mine,
All mine

So let this be a warning to all of you girls out there
If you see some guy with that gleam in his eyes
Well you'd better be prepared
Cos he loves Momma's Cookin'
And he loves his Momma's wine
So find a man who can understand
It'll make you feel so fine, so fine
So fine

I said damn yeah
I said damn yeah
I said damn your Momma's Cookin'
I say damn your Momma's wine
Cos I waited there
Every single day, but you wasted all my time

You wasted ... you wasted
You wasted all my lonely, lonely time
Oh no not your Momma, oh no not
Her wine
I said No No No No No!

Ain't It Strange?

I remember you told me that all gifts were holy
And I believed every word that you said
I trusted in truth as you do in your youth
Ain't it strange how it all slips away

Well I'm no pretender and I'll never surrender
To hatred and all that it brings
But you can learn wrong from right
Then forget when to fight
Ain't it strange how it all slips away

And I've been searching for reasons to rhyme
With the seasons
An I know that I've still far to go
But you have to be strong
Or you'll get shat upon
Ain't it strange how it all slips away

So please hear me now cos I'm happy and proud
To hold onto all I believe
So look back to those days
Don't just throw them away
Ain't it strange how it all slips away

Cos I remember you told me that all gifts were holy
And I believed every word that you said
I trusted in truth as you do in your youth
Ain't it strange how it all slips away.

Rosie.

Rosie sleeps without a man
She's 34 with an open door
Rosie learns to turn her key
It's another day at the factory
One day Rosie jumps out of bed
She's 35 and with a burning pride
Runs to the mirror and there she sees
She's older
Hang onto your dreams
Rosie steps out on the town
She sees a friend, so she laughs again
Rosie prays shell meet someone
To shield her from the days to come
Rosie girl you've got all you need
Your time has come
And life is so much fun
Times aren't as hard as they seem
But we're older
Hang onto your dreams
Rosie takes a joker home
She's knows he's fake but doesn't hesitate
Rosie calls me on the phone
To justify why she's still alone
One day Rosie jumps out of bed
She's 35 and with a burning pride
Runs to the mirror and there she sees
She's older, hang onto your dreams
Rosie's making changes now
Her chips are down
And she's no one's clown
But Rosie dont you hide away
Rebuild your life please don't delay
Cos Rosie girl you've got all you need

Your time has come
And life is so much fun
Times aren't as hard as they seem
But we're older
Hang onto your dreams
Rosie sleeps without a man
She's 34 with an open door
Rosie learns to turn her key
It's another day at the factory.

Full Circle.
Well it's a roundabout affair
Touching heart and touching soul
Followed you all over town
You never answer to my call
Saw you walking down the road
Another girl tucked in your arm
I just lost all self-control
I didn't mean her any harm
And now we've come full circle
Yes we've come full circle
It's been two weeks since that day
And I swear that I have paid
For the language that I used
And the sweet love that we made
But it's a roundabout affair
Touching heart and touching soul
Followed you all over town
You never answer to my call
And I have never met a man
Who balanced women like you can
Was she cold or just too plain
And is that why you call again?
And now we've come full circle
Yes we've full circle
But it's a roundabout affair
Touching heart and touching soul
Followed you all over town
You never answer to my call.

Come To Me.
Picture this darling it's a warm day in June
Shine all your lights
And make way for that silver moon
You can come to me
I will stay with you
You can come to me
Come to me
You can come to me

Don't hesitate while there's a fire burning here
Don't make me wait
I'm freezing all year
You can come to me
And I will stay with you
You can come to me
Come to me
You can come to me

You make it feel like summers here again....

Lay down your arms
There's no room for anger here
Surrender your charms
The night is ours

Come and take the wheel
You can come to me
And I will stay with you
You can come to me
Come to me
You can come to me

So picture this darling
It's a warm day in June
Shine all your lights and make way
For that silver moon.

Hello Daydream.

Verse 1:
Hello Daydream I know you
My dear Daydream,
What the hell am I gonna do?
I'm so restless, I have tried
Walked these rooms now,
Won't you give me piece of mind?
Just a little piece of mind
(Cos I) won't sleep before the dawn
(But I) won't weep now you're gone

Verse 2:
Life's for learning, that's no lie
Loving you has been my one and only crime
(But) I've got power, that's my own
Leave you hanging when you call me on the phone
Won't you call me on the phone?
(Cos I) won't sleep before the dawn
(But I) won't weep now you're gone

Well I've heard too much of your lovers and your lies
How breaking hearts is one thing you've always despised
But when you hold me all those words just fade away
Yeah, when you hold me I can't hear a word they say

Verse 3:
So it's one for sorrow and it's two for joy
I'll stay here and dream of every single ploy
Keep you darlin', keep you near
Love won't hide this time, it'll never disappear
Let it never disappear
(Cos I) won't sleep before the dawn
(But I) won't weep now you're gone

Hello Daydream I know you
My dear daydream, what the hell am I gonna do?

I Will Not Walk Behind.
Thoughts in my bed again
Words that don't come out
You're in my head again
And this time there is no doubt
That I'm thankful but I will not walk the line

When you had your chances
And then you took your time
To come home at night and to
To make our stories rhyme
So I will not stay, (No!) I will not walk behind

We're in our bed again
For some afternoon delight
I feel that dread again,
I've got to turn off this light
When the love you make leaves you stranded in the cold
It's time to move on up and take nothing you can't hold
You're always angry, why?
When you used to be so kind
So I will not stay, no I will not walk behind

Yes it's over now and I will not waste your time.

Short And Sweet.
It's hard to be honest
To reveal the real you
When you write your lines to rhyme
While you file and sharpen
And remove all the waste

Sometimes she just shows up
And jumps all the queues
Blatant and coarse or abrupt
But mostly we hide
Seeking perfection has its own risks

When you dress it up fancy
You lose all the heart
Seek to please and it's already gone
Don't try too hard and it's already there
The foundations of your perfect song.

Modern Life.

What you say and what you do
And how you share your point of view
Is all that matters today
What you eat and how you pray
And if you waste your days away
Someone will always judge you

So take a trip out to the shore
Forgot their jaded metaphors
The breeze will dance to your tune
Some mistakes you can't erase
We learn to live another day
The good light can always shine through

Modern life is up for sale
Go shopping for your fucking kale
I don't want to keep up with you

Modern life is triggered rage
I won't be coming out to play
A camera is all you look through.

I Write This Song For Everyone.
I write this song for everyone
Who's ever lost their somebody to love
You look around and there's no one there
Search for clues from up above

I write this song for everyone
Who's hanging on just much as they can
You can't prepare when you're unaware
That you'll need a change of plan

Nobody told me it could hurt like this
Tears that never run dry
Nobody warned me there'd be days like this
And that I'd question …why oh why?

I write this song for everyone
Who's ever sunk just before they could swim
You build a wall to protect yourself
And now you can't let anyone in

Nobody told me it could hurt like this

Tears that never run dry

Nobody warned me there'd be days like this

And that I'd question… why
Oh why?

I'll close my song now for everyone
Now I feel better in so many ways
So share your load before it all explodes
We're all the same

At the end of the end of the day
We're all the same at the end of the day.

Getting Old.
The world is more forthcoming
When you have beautiful limbs
Skin that is sure fire
And a smile that isn't drawn on
It wants to hear more
And to teach you to dance
Show you off to the chosen
Vacuum pack your youth
No you don't know what you've got
Til it's gone

Pity me as I reflect
Full of self-doubt and refute
My hair a thin veil of sacrifice
I gave my heart to the fire of
Longing and lust
Now invisible and out of the way
All packed up
No disturbance necessary.

Daze Nineteen.

Gave the coffee maker
A right seeing to!
Descaled and shining
With the urge to oblige
My every whim or fancy
For ever she rests by my side

Write what you feel
Write what you see!
Forever looking for ample opportunities
Buckle up, Baby we're gonna go far
You with that voice me with this smile
Gonna write me a classic on this here guitar

This staying home palaver
It might do us all in
Thank God I have words
To address at my whim
I'm eating and smoking
And playing around
Now finally a member of that inclusive In Crowd

30 Years On.
So that much too young girl
You fucked in more ways than one
Has sprouted wings and flown
Out of your grasp
Over the hills
To find her own space
Away from your hold
Rocking the boat to and fro

Did it make you feel uneasy
With that time on your hands?
Did it make you wonder why?
Looking to blame anyone else
For the fortress of unhappiness you built
Protecting your interests with foul language
And accusations

Then you went for your children
It was all their fault too
For leaving with "her"
No acceptable answer I am afraid
Twisted and nasty you even hated yourself
Eventually but not quick enough

So that is the bitter tale
Of a marriage far too young
17 and & mother
I loved my baby and cooking dinner with
Comfort and care to those who called
But the iceberg was you
The grey clouds your moods
I flinched as your key turned
The end was apparent even then

Before Verbal and Emotional
Abuse was even a thing
Before I had the courage to flee.

Fortune's Daughter.
Fortune's Daughter
With her Joie de Vivre
Rides high in her carriage today
Perfectly groomed, that smile, her face
Three hours of make-up
Not a hair out of place

Money never haunts her
She's got adequate supply
Momma's little angel
Poppa's joy and pride

Fortune's Daughter
With her corkscrew curls
Rides high in her carriage today
Born to excel, a privilege for few
Unlike the other brave girls I knew
She could have inspired or taught:
A fair trade
But shopping for boys
Was the decision she made

Money never haunts her
She's got adequate supply
Momma's little angel
Poppa's joy and pride
Fortunes Daughter
Has fallen behind
Rides high in her carriage today
She seeks your approval at every turn
Reassured by her beauty and charm
Measures boys for their value
Her girls for their clothes

No one to rescue, no one to harm
Hollow empty feelings can cause great alarm
Money never haunts her
She's got adequate supply
Momma's little angel
Poppa's joy and pride

Fortune's Daughter
Addictions appeased
Rides high in her carriage today
Takes off her clothes
And jumps right in
The water is shallow but she feels no cold
No one saw through her thin veneer
As she partied with her freedom
Yet felt so alone

Her cries for help were always unheard
Her reasons to us, felt trite and absurd
To have so much yet never be full
To never value her place, or to learn how to serve

Money never haunts her
She's got adequate supply
Momma's little angel
Poppa's joy and pride.

Writer's Whim.
Do you know what this passion is?
A love affair of words and tense
Of reference and refrain
Images floating by
Trying to capture the picture in a moment
To remember how it felt
It's texture or its warmth
It's sharpness or its mound;
The contrast.

Where will this lead?
Perhaps god already knows
I'm not that important.
But it's brought me some peace
And a reason to believe
In a time when faith is foolish
Old songs re-sung. New ones being built
.. Glory.

Acknowledgements –

I fell in love with words at a very early age. By 4 I was swooning after hearing George Harrison sing, "let me whisper in your ear, say the words I long to hear." Then it was Judy Garland. And Sinatra. The raw emotion "I saw a man who danced with his wife in Chicago." Then came the multiple wonderful singer songwriters of the 60s and 70s and my heaven was made. I must admit to having a photographic memory for lyrics. Always so vital to me. I started songwriting at 30 and wrote my first poem at 59. I am now 60.Thrilled to be offered to publish this book. A huge shout out to Colin Meek.

Heidi April
2020

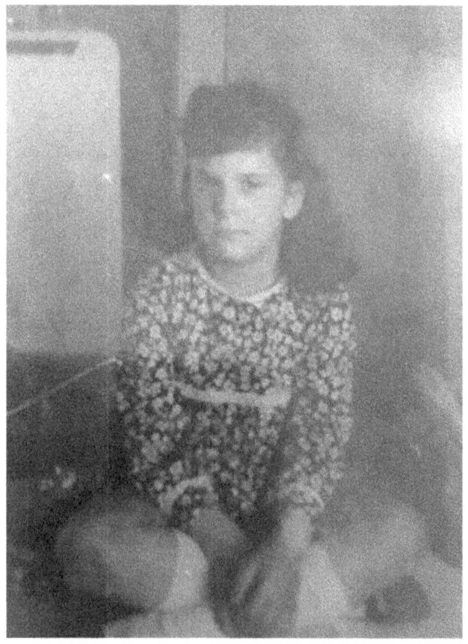